PCOS Diet For Type-2 Diabetes Patients

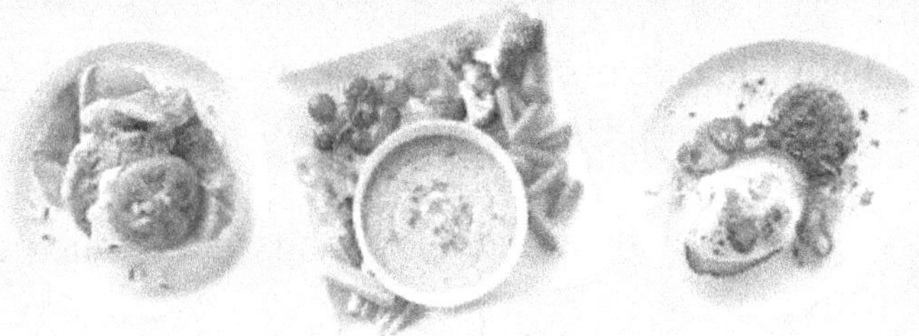

The Ultimate Guide To Managing PCOS And Type-2 Diabetes Through Diet With Meal Plans, Recipes And More

Dr Marcia Moss

Copyright © 2023 by Dr Marcia Moss.

The information provided in this book is for educational purposes and is not intended as a substitute for professional medical advice, diagnosis, or treatment. Always seek the advice of your physician or other qualified health provider with any questions you may have regarding a medical condition.

Thank You for Choosing Our Book

Embarking on the journey to a healthier lifestyle is a commendable decision, and we are genuinely grateful that you've chosen our book to guide you on this transformative path. To express our gratitude and enhance your experience with our book, we are committed to providing continuous support.

How to Get in Touch:

Should you encounter any challenges, have questions, or need clarification on any aspect of the book, we encourage you to reach out to us. Your feedback is invaluable, and we are here to assist you in making the most out of your journey to a healthier you.

Contact Email: drmarciamoss@gmail.com

TABLE OF CONTENTS

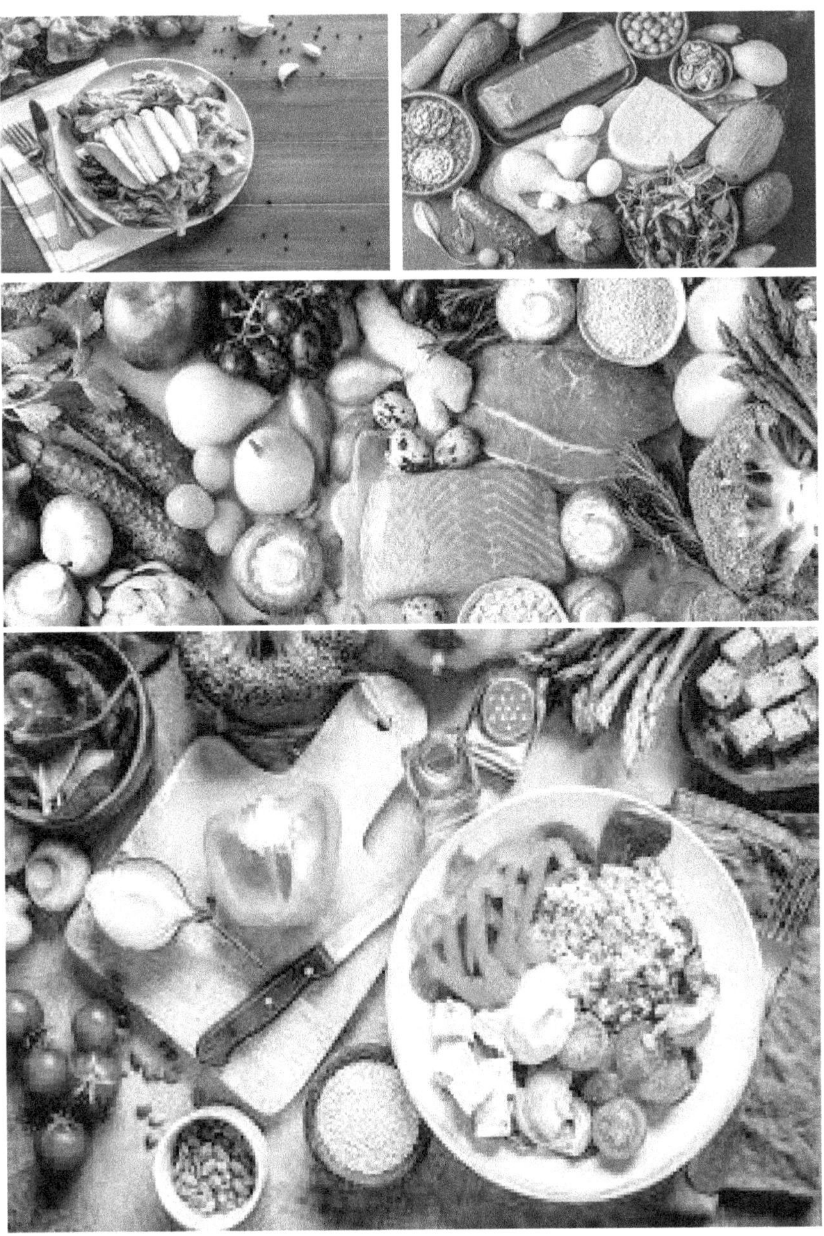

Introduction

Ever since 18-year-old Jane was diagnosed with PCOS and Type 2 Diabetes, she felt like she had lost control of her life. Her periods were irregular, her energy levels were low, and she struggled to lose weight. She felt like she was constantly at war with her own body.

But Jane didn't give up. She knew that there had to be a way to manage her conditions and live a healthy, happy life. She started researching and found a wealth of information about PCOS and Type 2 Diabetes. She learned that diet played a major role in managing these conditions.

Jane decided to make a change. She started eating a PCOS and Type 2 Diabetes-friendly diet, which included plenty of fruits, vegetables, whole grains, and lean protein. She also reduced her intake of processed foods, sugary drinks, and unhealthy fats.

At first, it was difficult for Jane to stick to her new diet. She was used to eating unhealthy foods, and she missed them. But she persevered, and soon she started to see results. Her periods became regular, her energy levels increased, and she started to lose weight.

Jane's health journey was not easy, but it was worth it. She learned that she could manage her conditions and live a healthy, happy life. She is now an inspiration to others who are struggling with PCOS and Type 2 Diabetes.

If you're ready to take control of your health and your life, then this book is for you. It will provide you with the information and support you need to make a positive change.

Chapter 1: Understanding PCOS and Type 2 Diabetes

Welcome to   your journey towards a healthier and more balanced life with PCOS and Type 2 diabetes. This chapter aims to equip you with a comprehensive understanding of these conditions and how they interrelate, paving the path for effective management through dietary interventions..

PCOS: Unveiling the Mystery

Polycystic Ovary Syndrome (PCOS) affects approximately 1 in 10 women of childbearing age, making it a prevalent condition. It is characterized by a hormonal imbalance, often leading to irregular periods, excess androgen (male hormone) levels, and the development of small cysts on the ovaries. These cysts, while benign, contribute to the hormonal imbalance and can cause a range of symptoms, including:

- Irregular periods or amenorrhea (absence of periods)

- Excess facial and body hair

- Acne

- Male pattern baldness

- Weight gain or difficulty losing weight

- Insulin resistance

- Infertility

Type 2 Diabetes: Understanding the Blood Sugar Rollercoaster

Type 2 diabetes, a chronic condition affecting how your body uses insulin, impacts millions of individuals worldwide. In simple terms, your body either doesn't produce enough insulin or doesn't use it effectively, leading to high blood sugar levels. These elevated levels, if left unchecked, can lead to serious health complications, such as:

- Heart disease

- Stroke

- Kidney disease

- Nerve damage

- Vision problems

The Intricate Connection: How PCOS and Type 2 Diabetes Collaborate

A significant number of women with PCOS develop insulin resistance, a condition where your body struggles to use insulin effectively. This resistance is a key factor in the development of Type 2 diabetes. Additionally, the hormonal imbalance associated with PCOS can further contribute to insulin resistance and exacerbate the challenges of managing blood sugar levels.

Diet: Your Powerful Tool for Managing Both Conditions

Fortunately, even amidst the complexities of PCOS and Type 2 diabetes, there's one powerful tool you hold in your own hands: diet. Implementing a healthy eating plan can significantly improve your condition and reduce the risk of complications. This is because food directly affects your blood sugar levels, insulin sensitivity, and overall health.

Diving Deeper: Key Nutrients for Management

Understanding the specific nutrients that support your health and combat the effects of PCOS and Type 2 diabetes is crucial. Here are some key nutrients to prioritize:

- **Fiber:** This dietary hero slows down the digestion process, preventing blood sugar spikes and promoting satiety.

- **Magnesium:** This mineral helps your body use insulin more effectively.

- **Chromium:** This trace mineral enhances insulin sensitivity and may improve blood sugar control.

- **Healthy fats:** Unsaturated fats, found in nuts, seeds, and avocado, promote satiety and improve insulin sensitivity.

Foods to Limit or Avoid

While incorporating essential nutrients is crucial, it's equally important to be mindful of foods that can exacerbate your condition. Here are some foods to limit or avoid:

- **Refined carbohydrates:** White bread, pasta, pastries, and sugary drinks cause rapid blood sugar spikes and contribute to insulin resistance.

- **Sugary foods and drinks**: These empty calories contribute to weight gain and worsen insulin resistance.

- **Processed meats:** These meats are often high in saturated fat, which can negatively impact your health.

- **Saturated and trans fats:** Found in fried foods and processed foods, these fats contribute to inflammation and insulin resistance.

Remember, understanding PCOS and Type 2 diabetes is the first step towards effective management. By adopting a healthy eating plan, you can gain control of your condition, improve your overall well-being, and embark on a journey towards a healthier and more fulfilling life. This chapter serves as a foundation for your journey, providing a solid understanding and empowering you to take charge of your health.

Chapter 2: Implementing the PCOS and Type 2 Diabetes Diet

Now that you possess a firm understanding of PCOS and Type 2 diabetes, it's time to translate knowledge into action. This chapter will guide you through implementing the dietary changes essential for managing both conditions effectively.

Building Balanced Meal Plans: A Blueprint for Success

Creating balanced meal plans is the cornerstone of effectively managing PCOS and Type 2 diabetes. These plans should prioritize:

- **Balanced macronutrients:** Aim for a plate composition that includes roughly half non-starchy vegetables, a quarter lean protein, and a quarter whole grains or healthy fats.

- **Regular meals and snacks**: Eating every 3-4 hours helps regulate blood sugar levels and prevent overeating at larger meals.

- **Portion control:** Mindful eating and understanding appropriate portion sizes are crucial for weight management, a key factor in managing both conditions.

- **Variety:** Incorporating a wide range of colorful fruits and vegetables ensures you receive essential vitamins, minerals, and antioxidants.

Sample Meal Plans for Different Needs:

No two individuals are exactly alike, and your dietary needs will depend on factors like age, activity level, and individual preferences. This section provides sample meal plans for various scenarios to help you tailor your diet to your specific needs

Sample Meal Plan 1: Standard PCOS and Type 2 Diabetes

- **Breakfast**: Greek yogurt with berries and chia seeds

- **Lunch:** Grilled chicken salad with whole-wheat pita bread

- **Dinner:** Salmon with roasted vegetables and brown rice

- **Snacks:** Fruits and nuts, vegetable sticks with hummus

Sample Meal Plan 2: Vegetarian PCOS and Type 2 Diabetes

- **Breakfast:** Oatmeal with fruit and nuts

- **Lunch:** Lentil soup with whole-grain bread

- **Dinner:** Tofu stir-fry with brown rice

- **Snacks**: Carrot sticks with cottage cheese, vegetable sticks with guacamole

Sample Meal Plan 3: Pre-diabetes with PCOS

- **Breakfast:** Whole-wheat toast with avocado and egg

- **Lunch:** Turkey sandwich on whole-wheat bread with side salad

- **Dinner:** Chicken breast with quinoa and roasted Brussels sprouts

- **Snacks:** Apple slices with almond butter, low-fat yogurt with mixed berries

- **Breakfast:** Gluten-free oatmeal with berries and chia seeds

- **Lunch:** Quinoa salad with grilled chicken or tofu

- **Dinner:** Baked cod with roasted sweet potatoes and green beans

- **Snack:** Gluten-free crackers with hummus

Shopping for a PCOS and Type 2 Diabetes Diet:

Planning your grocery shopping trips is essential for success. Here are some tips:

- **Read food labels carefully:** Pay attention to serving sizes, carbohydrates, and sugar content.

- **Focus on whole foods:** Opt for fresh fruits and vegetables, whole grains, lean protein sources, and healthy fats.

- **Limit processed foods**: Avoid sugary drinks, packaged snacks, and processed meats.

- **Plan your meals and snacks:** Make a list of needed ingredients to avoid impulse purchases.

- **Utilize frozen and canned options:** These can be convenient and healthy choices if selected wisely.

Cooking Tips and Techniques: Unleash Your Inner Chef

Cooking can be a fun and rewarding experience, especially when preparing delicious and healthy meals that support your well-being. Here are some tips to get you started:

- **Emphasize grilling, baking, and steaming:** These cooking methods are healthier alternatives to frying.

- **Experiment with spices and herbs**: These can add flavor without adding unhealthy fats or sugars.

- **Prepare meals in advance:** This saves time and ensures healthy options are readily available.

- **Involve family and friends:** Cooking together can be a fun and educational experience for everyone.

Overcoming Challenges and Staying Motivated: Maintaining Your Path

Implementing dietary changes can be challenging at times, but remember, you're not alone. Here are some strategies to overcome obstacles and stay motivated:

- **Set realistic goals:** Start with small, achievable changes and gradually build upon them.

- **Celebrate your successes**: Acknowledge and reward yourself for reaching your goals.

- **Find a support system:** Connect with friends, family, or online communities for encouragement.

- **Seek professional guidance:** Reach out to a registered dietitian or nutritionist for individualized guidance.

- **Don't give up:** Remember, progress takes time and effort. Be kind to yourself and focus on the long-term benefits.

Chapter 3: Delicious Recipes

Breakfast Recipes

1. Greek Yogurt Parfait with Berries and Almonds

- Ingredients:

- 1 cup Greek yogurt

- 1/2 cup mixed berries (strawberries, blueberries, raspberries)

- 1 tablespoon chia seeds

- 1 tablespoon slivered almonds

Instructions:

1. In a glass or bowl, layer Greek yogurt, mixed berries, chia seeds, and slivered almonds.

2. Repeat the layers.

3. Serve chilled.

- Serving Size: 1 parfait

- **Nutritional Information:**

  - Calories: 300

  - Protein: 20g

  - Carbohydrates: 30g

  - Fat: 12g

  - Fiber: 8g

2. Vegetarian Omelette with Spinach and Feta

- **Ingredients:**

  - 2 large eggs

  - 1/2 cup fresh spinach, chopped

  - 2 tablespoons feta cheese, crumbled

  - Salt and pepper to taste

  - 1 teaspoon olive oil

Instructions:

1. Whisk eggs in a bowl and season with salt and pepper.

2. Heat olive oil in a pan, add spinach and sauté until wilted.

3. Pour whisked eggs over the spinach, add feta, and cook until eggs are set.

4. Fold the omelette and serve.

-

Serving Size: 1 omelette

- Nutritional Information:

- Calories: 280

- Protein: 18g

- Carbohydrates: 3g

- Fat: 22g

- Fiber: 1g

3. Chia Seed Pudding with Mango

- Ingredients:

- 2 tablespoons chia seeds

- 1/2 cup unsweetened almond milk

- 1/2 teaspoon vanilla extract

- 1/2 cup diced mango

- Instructions:

1. Mix chia seeds, almond milk, and vanilla extract in a bowl.

2. Refrigerate for at least 2 hours or overnight until it thickens.

3. Top with diced mango before serving.

- Serving Size: 1 serving

- Nutritional Information:

- Calories: 180

- Protein: 5g

- Carbohydrates: 25g

- Fat: 8g

- Fiber: 10g

4. Whole Wheat Toast with Avocado and Poached Egg

- Ingredients:

- 1 slice whole wheat bread

- 1/2 avocado, mashed

- 1 poached egg

- Salt and pepper to taste

- Instructions:

1. Toast the whole wheat bread.

2. Spread mashed avocado on the toast.

3. Top with a poached egg and season with salt and pepper.

- Serving Size: 1 serving

- Nutritional Information:

- Calories: 250

- Protein: 12g

- Carbohydrates: 20g

- Fat: 15g

- Fiber: 8g

5. Mixed Berry Smoothie Bowl

- Ingredients:

- 1 cup mixed berries (strawberries, blueberries, raspberries)

- 1/2 banana

- 1/2 cup Greek yogurt

- 1 tablespoon chia seeds

- Ice cubes (optional)

- Instructions:

1. Blend mixed berries, banana, Greek yogurt, and chia seeds until smooth.

2. Pour into a bowl and top with additional berries.

- Serving Size: 1 bowl

- Nutritional Information:

- Calories: 220

- Protein: 15g

- Carbohydrates: 35g

- Fat: 5g

- Fiber: 8g

6. Quinoa Breakfast Bowl with Almond Butter

- Ingredients:

- 1/2 cup cooked quinoa

- 1/2 banana, sliced

- 1 tablespoon almond butter

- 1 tablespoon chopped nuts (almonds, walnuts)

- Instructions:

1. Mix cooked quinoa with banana slices.

2. Drizzle with almond butter and sprinkle chopped nuts on top.

- Serving Size: 1 serving

- Nutritional Information:

-   Calories: 300

-   Protein: 10g

-   Carbohydrates: 40g

-   Fat: 12g

-   Fiber: 5g

7. Gluten-Free Pancakes with Berries

- Ingredients:

- 1/2 cup gluten-free pancake mix

- 1/3 cup almond milk

- 1 egg

- 1/2 cup mixed berries

- Instructions:

1. Mix pancake mix, almond milk, and egg until well combined.

2. Cook pancakes on a griddle until golden brown.

3. Top with mixed berries.

- Serving Size: 2 pancakes

- Nutritional Information:

- Calories: 250

- Protein: 8g

- Carbohydrates: 35g

- Fat: 8g

- Fiber: 5g

8. Egg Muffins with Spinach and Tomatoes

- Ingredients:

- 2 large eggs

- 1/2 cup fresh spinach, chopped

- 1/4 cup cherry tomatoes, diced

- Salt and pepper to taste

- Instructions:

1. Preheat the oven to 350°F (175°C).

2. Whisk the eggs and season them with salt and pepper.

3. Mix in chopped spinach and diced tomatoes.

4. Pour the mixture into muffin cups and bake for 15-20 minutes.

- Serving Size: 2 muffins

- Nutritional Information:

- Calories: 200

- Protein: 14g

- Carbohydrates: 5g

- Fat: 15g

- Fiber: 2g

9. Sweet Potato Hash with Turkey Sausage

- Ingredients:

- 1 medium sweet potato, grated

- 2 turkey sausage links, sliced

- 1/2 bell pepper, diced

- 1/4 onion, diced

- 1 tablespoon olive oil

- Instructions:

1. Heat olive oil in a pan and sauté onion, bell pepper, and turkey sausage.

2. Add grated sweet potato and cook until everything is tender.

- Serving Size: 1 serving

- Nutritional Information:

- Calories: 300

- Protein: 15g

- Carbohydrates: 30g

- Fat: 15g

- Fiber: 5g

10. Avocado and Berry Smoothie

- Ingredients:

- 1/2 avocado

- 1/2 cup mixed berries (strawberries, blueberries, raspberries)

- 1 cup unsweetened almond milk

- 1 tablespoon chia seeds

- Instructions:

1. Blend avocado, mixed berries, almond milk, and chia seeds until smooth.

2. Pour into a glass and serve.

- Serving Size: 1 serving

- **Nutritional Information:**

  - Calories: 280

  - Protein: 5g

  - Carbohydrates: 25g

  - Fat: 18g

  - Fiber: 10g

Lunch Recipes

1. Grilled Chicken Salad with Quinoa and Avocado

- Ingredients:

- 4 oz grilled chicken breast

- 1 cup cooked quinoa

- Mixed salad greens

- 1/2 avocado, sliced

- Cherry tomatoes, halved

- Olive oil and balsamic vinegar dressing

- Instructions:

1. Season and grill the chicken breast.

2. Mix cooked quinoa, salad greens, avocado slices, and cherry tomatoes.

3. Top with grilled chicken and drizzle with olive oil and balsamic vinegar.

- Serving Size: 1 serving

- Nutritional Information:

    - Calories: 400

    - Protein: 30g

    - Carbohydrates: 30g

    - Fat: 18g

    - Fiber: 8g

2. Vegetarian Quinoa Bowl with Chickpeas and Roasted Vegetables

- **Ingredients:**

  - 1 cup cooked quinoa

  - 1/2 cup chickpeas, drained and rinsed

  - Mixed roasted vegetables (zucchini, bell peppers, cherry tomatoes)

  - Feta cheese, crumbled

  - Olive oil and lemon dressing

- **Instructions:**

1. Roast vegetables in olive oil until tender.

2. Mix cooked quinoa, chickpeas, and roasted vegetables.

3. Top with crumbled feta and Drizzle with a dressing of olive oil and lemon.

- Serving Size: 1 serving

- Nutritional Information:

- Calories: 380

- Protein: 15g

- Carbohydrates: 50g

- Fat: 15g

- Fiber: 10g

3. Salmon and Asparagus Foil Pack

- Ingredients:

- 4 oz salmon fillet

- Asparagus spears

- Lemon slices

- Fresh dill

- Olive oil

- Salt and pepper

- Instructions:

1. Place salmon on a foil sheet, surround with asparagus.

2. Drizzle with olive oil, add lemon slices and fresh dill.

3. Seal the foil and bake until salmon is cooked.

- Serving Size: 1 serving

- **Nutritional Information:**

    -   Calories: 350

    -   Protein: 25g

    -   Carbohydrates: 10g

    -   Fat: 22g

    -   Fiber: 5g

4. Vegetable and Lentil Soup

- Ingredients:

- 1 cup lentils, rinsed

- Mixed vegetables (carrots, celery, onion)

- Low-sodium vegetable broth

- Herbs and spices (thyme, bay leaves)

- Salt and pepper

- Instructions:

1. Cook lentils in vegetable broth with mixed vegetables and herbs.

2. Season with salt and pepper.

3. Simmer until lentils are tender.

- Serving Size: 1 serving

- Nutritional Information:

- Calories: 300

- Protein: 18g

- Carbohydrates: 50g

- Fat: 2g

- Fiber: 15g

5. Tofu Stir-Fry with Broccoli and Brown Rice

- Ingredients:

- 1 cup firm tofu, cubed

- Broccoli florets

- Carrots, sliced

- Brown rice, cooked

- Low-sodium soy sauce

- Sesame oil

- Instructions:

1. Stir-fry tofu, broccoli, and carrots in sesame oil.

2. Add cooked brown rice and soy sauce.

3. Cook until vegetables are tender.

- Serving Size: 1 serving

- Nutritional Information:

- Calories: 320

- Protein: 15g

- Carbohydrates: 45g

- Fat: 10g

- Fiber: 8g

6. Turkey and Quinoa Stuffed Bell Peppers

- Ingredients:

- Bell peppers, halved

- Ground turkey

- Cooked quinoa

- Black beans, drained and rinsed

- Tomato sauce

- Mexican seasoning blend

- Instructions:

1. Brown ground turkey, mix with cooked quinoa, black beans, and seasoning.

2. Stuff bell peppers with the mixture.

3. Bake until peppers are tender.

- Serving Size: 2 pepper halves

- **Nutritional Information:**

  - Calories: 380

  - Protein: 25g

  - Carbohydrates: 40g

  - Fat: 15g

  - Fiber: 10g

7. Chicken and Quinoa Salad with Mango Salsa

- Ingredients:

- Grilled chicken breast, sliced

- 1 cup cooked quinoa

- Mixed salad greens

- Mango salsa (mango, red onion, cilantro)

- Lime vinaigrette

- Instructions:

1. Mix cooked quinoa, salad greens, and sliced grilled chicken.

2. Top with mango salsa and drizzle with lime vinaigrette.

- Serving Size: 1 serving

- **Nutritional Information:**

- Calories: 400

- Protein: 30g

- Carbohydrates: 40g

- Fat: 15g

- Fiber: 8g

8. Eggplant and Chickpea Curry

- Ingredients:

- Eggplant, cubed

- Chickpeas, drained and rinsed

- Tomato sauce

- Curry spices (cumin, coriander, turmeric)

- Coconut milk

- Fresh cilantro

- **Instructions:**

1. Cook eggplant and chickpeas in tomato sauce and curry spices.

2. Stir in coconut milk and simmer until flavors meld.

3. Garnish with fresh cilantro.

- Serving Size: 1 serving

- **Nutritional Information:**

- Calories: 340

- Protein: 12g

- Carbohydrates: 45g

- Fat: 15g

- Fiber: 12g

9. Baked Cod with Quinoa and Roasted Vegetables

- Ingredients:

- Cod fillet

- 1 cup cooked quinoa

- Mixed roasted vegetables (zucchini, cherry tomatoes, bell peppers)

- Lemon wedges

- Olive oil

- Instructions:

1. Season cod with olive oil, salt, and pepper.

2. Bake until fish is cooked.

3. Serve over cooked quinoa and roasted vegetables.

- Serving Size: 1 serving

- Nutritional Information:

- Calories: 320

- Protein: 30g

- Carbohydrates: 30g

- Fat: 10g

- Fiber: 8g

10. Mediterranean Chickpea Salad

- Ingredients:

- Chickpeas, drained and rinsed

- Cucumber, diced

- Cherry tomatoes, halved

- Kalamata olives, sliced

- Feta cheese, crumbled

- Olive oil and lemon dressing

- Instructions:

1. Combine chickpeas, cucumber, tomatoes, olives, and feta in a bowl.

2. Drizzle with olive oil and lemon dressing.

- Serving Size: 1 serving

- Nutritional Information:

- Calories: 340

- Protein: 15g

- Carbohydrates: 35g

- Fat: 18g

- Fiber: 10g

Dinner Recipes

1. Salmon with Quinoa and Roasted Vegetables

- Ingredients:

- 6 oz salmon fillet

- 1/2 cup cooked quinoa

- Mixed roasted vegetables (asparagus, bell peppers, cherry tomatoes)

- Lemon wedges

- Olive oil

- Instructions:

1. Season salmon with olive oil, salt, and pepper.

2. Bake until salmon is cooked.

3. Serve over a bed of cooked quinoa and roasted vegetables.

- Serving Size: 1 serving

- **Nutritional Information:**

    - Calories: 400

    - Protein: 30g

    - Carbohydrates: 30g

    - Fat: 18g

    - Fiber: 8g

2. Vegetarian Stir-Fried Tofu with Broccoli and Brown Rice

- Ingredients:

- 1 cup firm tofu, cubed

- Broccoli florets

- Carrots, sliced

- Brown rice, cooked

- Low-sodium soy sauce

- Sesame oil

- Instructions:

1. Stir-fry tofu, broccoli, and carrots in sesame oil.

2. Add cooked brown rice and soy sauce.

3. Cook until vegetables are tender.

- Serving Size: 1 serving

- Nutritional Information:

- Calories: 340

- Protein: 15g

- Carbohydrates: 45g

- Fat: 10g

- Fiber: 8g

3. Grilled Chicken Breast with Sweet Potato Mash and Steamed Asparagus

- Ingredients:

- 6 oz grilled chicken breast

- 1 medium sweet potato, mashed

- Steamed asparagus spears

- Olive oil

- Garlic powder and paprika

- Instructions:

- Grill chicken breast with olive oil, garlic powder, and paprika.

- Steam asparagus and serve alongside sweet potato mash.

- Serving Size: 1 serving

- Nutritional Information:

- Calories: 380

- Protein: 30g

- Carbohydrates: 35g

- Fat: 15g

- Fiber: 8g

4. Turkey and Vegetable Quinoa Bowl

- Ingredients:

- Ground turkey

- Mixed vegetables (including bell peppers, zucchini, and cherry tomatoes).

- 1 cup cooked quinoa

- Olive oil

- Italian seasoning

- Instructions:

1. Brown ground turkey with olive oil and Italian seasoning.

2. Add mixed vegetables and cook until tender.

3. Serve over cooked quinoa.

- Serving Size: 1 serving

- **Nutritional Information:**

  - Calories: 350

  - Protein: 25g

  - Carbohydrates: 35g

  - Fat: 15g

  - Fiber: 8g

5. Baked Cod with Lemon-Dill Sauce and Steamed Green Beans

- **Ingredients:**

  - Cod fillet

  - Fresh lemon juice

  - Fresh dill, chopped

  - Olive oil

  - Steamed green beans

- Instructions:

1. Season cod with olive oil, lemon juice, and chopped dill.

2. Bake until fish is cooked.

3. Serve with steamed green beans.

- Serving Size: 1 serving

- Nutritional Information:

- Calories: 320

- Protein: 30g

- Carbohydrates: 15g

- Fat: 15g

- Fiber: 8g

6. Mushroom and Spinach Quiche with a Quinoa Crust

- Ingredients:

- 1 cup cooked quinoa

- Eggs

- Spinach, chopped

- Mushrooms, sliced

- Low-fat cheese

- Milk (dairy or plant-based)

- Instructions:

1. Mix cooked quinoa with eggs and press into a pie dish.

2. Sauté mushrooms and spinach, then spread over the quinoa crust.

3. Pour a mixture of eggs and milk over the vegetables.

4. Top with low-fat cheese and bake until set.

- Serving Size: 1 slice

- **Nutritional Information:**

  - Calories: 300

  - Protein: 20g

  - Carbohydrates: 25g

  - Fat: 15g

  - Fiber: 5g

7. Lentil and Vegetable Curry with Cauliflower Rice

- **Ingredients:**

  - Lentils, cooked

  - Mixed vegetables (bell peppers, carrots, peas)

  - Tomato sauce

  - Curry spices (cumin, coriander, turmeric)

  - Cauliflower rice

- **Instructions:**

1. Cook lentils with mixed vegetables, tomato sauce, and curry spices.

2. Serve over cauliflower rice.

- Serving Size: 1 serving

- **Nutritional Information:**

- Calories: 320

- Protein: 18g

- Carbohydrates: 50g

- Fat: 2g

- Fiber: 15g

8. Chickpea and Spinach Stuffed Bell Peppers

- Ingredients:

- Bell peppers, halved

- Chickpeas, mashed

- Spinach, chopped

- Quinoa, cooked

- Tomato sauce

- Italian herbs

- Instructions:

1. Mix mashed chickpeas with chopped spinach, cooked quinoa, and tomato sauce.

2. Stuff bell peppers with the mixture.

3. Bake until peppers are tender.

- Serving Size: 2 pepper halves

- **Nutritional Information:**

  - Calories: 350

  - Protein: 15g

  - Carbohydrates: 40g

  - Fat: 12g

  - Fiber: 10g

9. Eggplant Lasagna with Ground Turkey and Zucchini

- **Ingredients:**

  - Eggplant, thinly sliced

  - Ground turkey

  - Zucchini, thinly sliced

  - Low-sugar marinara sauce

  - Low-fat ricotta cheese

- Instructions:

1. Brown ground turkey and mix with marinara sauce.

2. Layer eggplant slices, ground turkey mixture, zucchini slices, and ricotta cheese.

3. Bake until bubbly and golden.

- Serving Size: 1 serving

- Nutritional Information:

- Calories: 380

- Protein: 25g

- Carbohydrates: 30g

- Fat: 18g

- Fiber: 10g

10. Shrimp and Vegetable Skewers with Quinoa

- Ingredients:

- Shrimp, peeled and deveined

- Bell peppers, cherry tomatoes, red onion (for skewers)

- Olive oil

- Lemon juice

- Quinoa, cooked

- Instructions:

1. Thread shrimp and vegetables onto skewers.

2. Grill until shrimp are cooked.

3. Serve over a bed of cooked quinoa, drizzled with olive oil and lemon juice.

- Serving Size: 1 serving

- Nutritional Information:

  - Calories: 320

  - Protein: 25g

  - Carbohydrates: 30g

  - Fat: 12g

  - Fiber: 8g

Snacks and Sides Recipes

1. Greek Yogurt and Berry Parfait

- Ingredients:

-   1 cup Greek yogurt

-   Mixed berries (strawberries, raspberries, blueberries)

-   1 tablespoon chia seeds

-   1 tablespoon crushed nuts (almonds, walnuts)

- Instructions:

1. In a glass, layer Greek yogurt with mixed berries.

2. Sprinkle chia seeds and crushed nuts on top.

- Serving Size: 1 parfait

- Nutritional Information:

  - Calories: 200

  - Protein: 15g

  - Carbohydrates: 20g

  - Fat: 8g

  - Fibre: 5g

2. Vegetable Sticks with Hummus

- Ingredients:

-   Carrot, cucumber, and bell pepper sticks

-   Hummus for dipping

- Instructions:

1. Cut vegetables into sticks.

2. Serve with hummus for dipping.

- Serving Size: 1 serving

- **Nutritional Information:**

   - Calories: 100

   - Protein: 3g

   - Carbohydrates: 15g

   - Fat: 5g

   - Fiber: 6g

3. Hard-Boiled Eggs with Avocado

- Ingredients:

- Hard-boiled eggs

- 1/2 avocado, sliced

- Salt and pepper to taste

- Instructions:

1. Slice hard-boiled eggs and arrange on a plate.

2. Top with sliced avocado and season with salt and pepper.

- Serving Size: 2 eggs with 1/2 avocado

- Nutritional Information:

- Calories: 250

- Protein: 15g

- Carbohydrates: 12g

- Fat: 18g

- Fiber: 8g

Ingredients:

- Almonds, walnuts, pistachios, and cashews

- Dried cranberries or raisins

- Dark chocolate chips

Instructions:

1. Mix nuts and dried fruits in a bowl.

2. Add dark chocolate chips.

Serving Size: 1/4 cup

Nutritional Information:

- Calories: 150

- Protein: 5g

- Carbohydrates: 10g

- Fat: 10g

- Fiber: 3g

5. Edamame and Cherry Tomato Salad

- Ingredients:

- Edamame beans, cooked

- Cherry tomatoes, halved

- Fresh basil, chopped

- Balsamic vinaigrette

- Instructions:

1. Combine edamame, cherry tomatoes, and basil in a bowl.

2. Pour a bit of balsamic vinaigrette over the dish.

- Serving Size: 1 serving

- **Nutritional Information:**

  - Calories: 150

  - Protein: 10g

  - Carbohydrates: 15g

  - Fat: 7g

  - Fiber: 5g

6. Guacamole with Veggie Sticks

- **Ingredients:**

  - Avocado, mashed

  - Tomato, diced

  - Red onion, finely chopped

  - Lime juice

  - Salt and pepper

  - Carrot and cucumber sticks for dipping

- Instructions:

1. Mix mashed avocado, diced tomato, chopped red onion, lime juice, salt, and pepper.

2. Enjoy with carrot and cucumber slices.

- Serving Size: 1 serving

- Nutritional Information:

- Calories: 180

- Protein: 3g

- Carbohydrates: 15g

- Fat: 14g

- Fiber: 8g

7. Whole Grain Crackers with Smoked Salmon

- Ingredients:

- Whole grain crackers

- Smoked salmon slices

- Cream cheese (optional)

- Fresh dill for garnish

- Instructions:

1. Top whole grain crackers with smoked salmon.

2. Optional: add a small amount of cream cheese.

3. Garnish with fresh dill.

- Serving Size: 1 serving

- Nutritional Information:

- Calories: 180

- Protein: 10g

- Carbohydrates: 15g

- Fat: 8g

- Fiber: 3g

8. Caprese Salad Skewers

- Ingredients:

- -Cherry tomatoes

- Mozzarella balls

- Fresh basil leaves

- Balsamic glaze

- **Instructions:**

1. Thread cherry tomatoes, mozzarella balls, and basil leaves onto skewers.

2. Drizzle with balsamic glaze.

- Serving Size: 1 serving

- **Nutritional Information:**

- Calories: 150

- Protein: 8g

- Carbohydrates: 6g

- Fat: 10g

- Fiber: 1g

9. Baked Sweet Potato Fries

- Ingredients:

- Sweet potatoes, cut into fries

- Olive oil

- Paprika and garlic powder

- Greek yogurt for dipping

- Instructions:

1. Toss sweet potato fries with olive oil, paprika, and garlic powder.

2. Bake until crispy.

3. Serve with a side of Greek yogurt for dipping.

- Serving Size: 1 serving

- **Nutritional Information:**

  - Calories: 180

  - Protein: 4g

  - Carbohydrates: 30g

  - Fat: 6g

  - Fiber: 4g

Dessert Recipes

1. Baked Cinnamon Apples

- Ingredients:

- 2 medium-sized apples, cored and sliced

- 1 tablespoon melted coconut oil

- 1 teaspoon ground cinnamon

- 1 tablespoon chopped walnuts

- Instructions:

1. Preheat oven to 375°F (190°C).

2. Toss apple slices with melted coconut oil and cinnamon.

3. Bake in a single layer until apples are tender.

4. Add a finishing touch by sprinkling chopped walnuts just before serving.

- Serving Size: 1/2 cup

- Nutritional Information:

- Calories: 120

- Protein: 1g

- Carbohydrates: 20g

- Fat: 6g

- Fiber: 4g

3. Dark Chocolate-Dipped Strawberries

- Ingredients:

- Fresh strawberries, washed and dried

- Dark chocolate (70% cocoa or higher)

- Instructions:

1. Melt dark chocolate in a microwave or on a stovetop.

2. Dip each strawberry into the melted chocolate.

3. Place on a parchment paper-lined tray and let it cool until the chocolate hardens.

- Serving Size: 2 strawberries

- Nutritional Information:

- Calories: 60

- Protein: 1g

- Carbohydrates: 10g

- Fat: 3g

- Fiber: 2g

3. Chia Seed Pudding with Berries

- Ingredients:

- 2 tablespoons chia seeds

- 1/2 cup unsweetened almond milk

- 1/2 teaspoon vanilla extract

- 1/2 cup mixed berries

- Instructions:

1. Mix chia seeds, almond milk, and vanilla extract in a bowl.

2. Refrigerate for a minimum of 2 hours or leave overnight.

3. Finish by garnishing with mixed berries just before serving.

- Serving Size: 1/2 cup

- Nutritional Information:

- Calories: 100

- Protein: 3g

- Carbohydrates: 12g

- Fat: 5g

- Fiber: 7g

4. Banana and Almond Butter Bites

- Ingredients:

- 1 medium banana, sliced

- 2 tablespoons almond butter

- Chopped nuts (walnuts or almonds) for topping

- Instructions:

1. Spread almond butter on banana slices.

2. Sprinkle with chopped nuts.

- Serving Size: 1 serving

- Nutritional Information:

- Calories: 150

- Protein: 3g

- Carbohydrates: 18g

- Fat: 9g

- Fiber: 3g

Meal Prep Tips: Optimize Your Time and Eating Habits

Meal prepping offers a powerful way to save time, eat healthier, and manage food costs. Here are some tips to optimize your meal prep experience:

Planning and Preparation:

- **Schedule:** Dedicate specific days and time slots for prepping meals.

- **Plan your menu:** Include variety and consider your dietary needs and preferences.

- **Create a grocery list:** Stick to your list to avoid impulse purchases.

- Chop vegetables and portion out ingredients in advance.

Cooking and Storage:

- **Cook in batches:** Prepare larger quantities to enjoy leftovers throughout the week.

- **Use versatile ingredients:** Choose items that can be used in multiple dishes.

- **Embrace variety:** Cook different protein sources, grains, and vegetables to keep things interesting.

- **Store meals properly:** Use airtight containers and refrigerate or freeze depending on shelf life.

Tips and Tricks:

- **Utilize slow cookers and pressure cookers:** Simplify cooking and save time.

- **Make breakfast ahead:** Prepare overnight oats, breakfast burritos, or chia pudding.

- **Double recipes:** Freeze half for later enjoyment.

- **Pack lunches and snacks:** Avoid unhealthy temptations throughout the day.

- **Clean as you go:** Minimize post-prep cleanup.

- **Get creative:** Experiment with new recipes and flavors.

Benefits:
s

- Saves time and reduces stress

- Promotes healthier eating habits

- Helps with portion control

- Reduces food waste

- Saves money on groceries

By incorporating these tips, you can turn meal prep into a valuable tool for managing your diet and leading a healthier lifestyle.

Chapter 4: Beyond Diet: A Holistic Approach to Your Well-being

While diet plays a pivotal role in managing PCOS and Type 2 diabetes, it's only one piece of the puzzle. Embracing a comprehensive approach encompassing exercise, stress management, sleep hygiene, and strong support systems is crucial for optimizing your health and well-being.

Exercise and Physical Activity: Your Body's Natural Ally

Regular physical activity offers a multitude of benefits for individuals with PCOS and Type 2 diabetes. It:

- **Improves insulin sensitivity:** This allows your body to use insulin more effectively, leading to better blood sugar control.

- **Promotes weight management:** Exercise helps you burn calories and maintain a healthy weight, which is crucial for managing both conditions.

- **Reduces inflammation:** Chronic inflammation is a key factor in both PCOS and Type 2 diabetes, and exercise helps combat it.

- **Boosts mood and energy levels:** Physical activity releases endorphins, which improve mood and combat fatigue, common symptoms of both conditions.

Aim for at least 30 minutes of moderate-intensity exercise most days of the week. Choose activities you enjoy, such as brisk walking, swimming, dancing, or cycling. Start slowly and gradually increase the duration and intensity of your workouts as your fitness level improves.

Stress Management and Sleep Hygiene: Finding Inner Peace

Stress can negatively impact both PCOS and Type 2 diabetes, leading to higher blood sugar levels and worsening symptoms. Finding effective stress management techniques is essential for promoting overall well-being. Consider incorporating practices like:

- **Mindfulness meditation:** This practice helps focus your attention and cultivate inner peace.

- **Yoga:** This combines physical postures with breathing exercises and relaxation techniques.

- **Deep breathing exercises:** These simple exercises can help calm your mind and body.

- **Spending time in nature:** Connecting with nature has a powerful calming effect.

Adequate sleep is also crucial for managing both conditions. Aim for 7-8 hours of sleep each night. Establish a regular sleep schedule and create a relaxing bedtime routine.

Monitoring and Tracking Progress: Empowering Yourself with Knowledge

Tracking your progress is essential to stay motivated and adjust your approach as needed. Consider keeping a log of:

- **Blood sugar levels:** This helps you understand how different foods and activities affect your blood sugar.

- **Weight:** Monitor your weight and strive for healthy weight management.

- **Food intake:** Track your food intake to ensure you're adhering to your dietary plan.

- **Exercise:** Log your workouts to stay motivated and track your progress.

Building a Support System: Finding Strength in Connection

Surrounding yourself with supportive individuals can significantly impact your well-being. Consider joining a support group for individuals with PCOS and Type 2 diabetes. These groups offer a safe space to connect with others who understand your challenges and offer encouragement and advice.

Additionally, confide in close friends, family members, or a therapist. Having someone to listen and offer support can make a world of difference.

With dedication and the right tools, you can thrive and conquer the challenges of these conditions.

Chapter 5: Conclusion

Congratulations! You've learned a boatload about managing PCOS and Type 2 diabetes through diet, exercise, stress management, and more. Now, let's boil it down to the essentials for your empowered journey to better health:

Diet:

- Make whole foods your best friends: They help control blood sugar, manage weight, and boost overall well-being.

- Choose variety: Mix things up with fruits, vegetables, whole grains, lean protein, and healthy fats.

- Find what works for you: Experiment and discover delicious recipes that fit your taste and dietary needs.

Exercise:

- Move your body in ways you enjoy: Dancing, walking, swimming, whatever gets you moving!

- Start slow and gradually increase: Consistency is key, so find an activity you can stick with.

- Make it a team effort: Exercise with friends or join a group class for added motivation.

- Stress Management:

- Find your stress-busters: Meditation, yoga, spending time in nature – find what calms your mind and soul.

- Prioritize sleep: Aim for 7-8 hours of quality sleep each night for optimal health.

- Don't bottle things up: Talk to loved ones, a therapist, or join a support group for understanding and encouragement.

Progress Tracking:

- Monitor your blood sugar, weight, and other metrics: This helps you stay on track and adjust your approach as needed.

- Celebrate your victories: Every step forward is a win, so be proud of your progress!

Support System:

- Build your team: Surround yourself with supportive people who understand your journey.

- **Connect with others**: Join a support group or find friends who can share their experiences and offer encouragement.

- **Don't hesitate to ask for help:** Your healthcare team is there to guide and support you every step of the way.

Remember:

- This journey is about YOU.

- Embrace the ups and downs, celebrate your victories, and stay focused on a healthier, happier future.

- You got this!

28 day Meal planner

Guide to Using the 28-Day Meal Planner

Meals:
- Plan each week's breakfast, lunch, dinner, and snacks.
- Try new recipes for variety.

Grocery List:
- Check your kitchen before shopping.
- Customize the sample shopping list.
- Organize items by category.
- Stick to your list, avoid impulse buys.

Notes:
- Track your progress and jot down observations.
- Personalize the plan to suit your preferences.
- Record any recipe changes and portion adjustments.

Enjoy your 28-day journey!

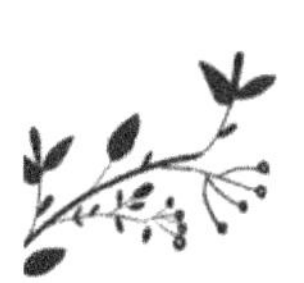

DAILY MEAL PLANNER

DATE: _______________________   M T W T F S S

BREAKFAST

GROCERY LIST

LUNCH

DINNER

NOTES

SNACKS

 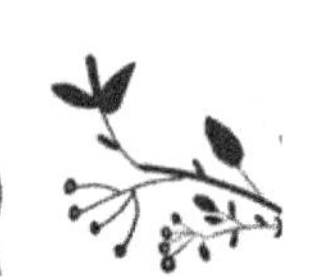

DAILY MEAL PLANNER

DATE ___________________________   M T W T F S S

BREAKFAST

GROCERY LIST

LUNCH

DINNER

NOTES

SNACKS

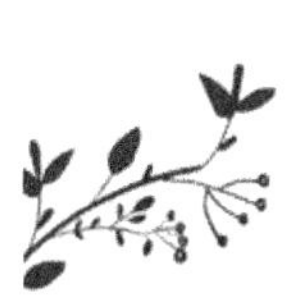 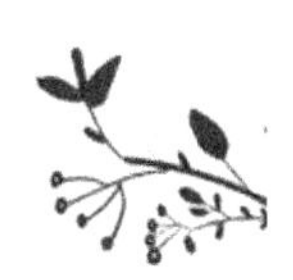

DAILY MEAL PLANNER

DATE: _______________________   M T W T F S S

BREAKFAST

GROCERY LIST

LUNCH

DINNER

NOTES

SNACKS

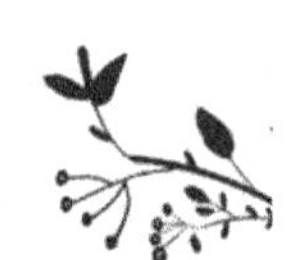

DAILY MEAL PLANNER

DATE: ___________________________   M T W T F S S

BREAKFAST

GROCERY LIST

LUNCH

DINNER

NOTES

SNACKS

DAILY MEAL PLANNER

DATE _______________________   M T W T F S S

BREAKFAST

LUNCH

DINNER

SNACKS

GROCERY LIST

NOTES

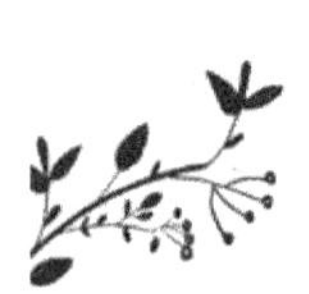 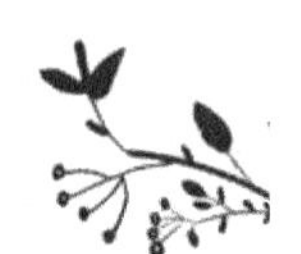

DAILY MEAL PLANNER

DATE: _______________________   M T W T F S S

BREAKFAST

GROCERY LIST

LUNCH

DINNER

NOTES

SNACKS

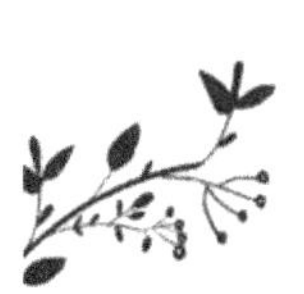

DAILY MEAL PLANNER

DATE: _______________________________   M T W T F S S

BREAKFAST

GROCERY LIST

LUNCH

DINNER

NOTES

SNACKS

 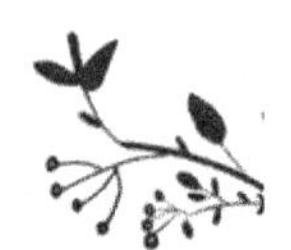

DAILY MEAL PLANNER

DATE _________________________   M T W T F S S

BREAKFAST

GROCERY LIST

LUNCH

DINNER

NOTES

SNACKS

 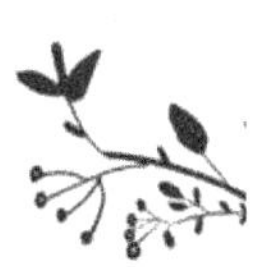

DAILY MEAL PLANNER

DATE: _______________________________   M T W T F S S

BREAKFAST

GROCERY LIST

LUNCH

DINNER

NOTES

SNACKS

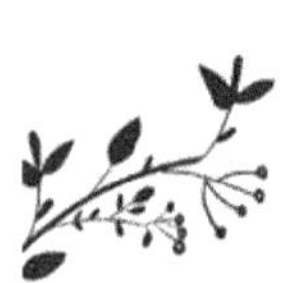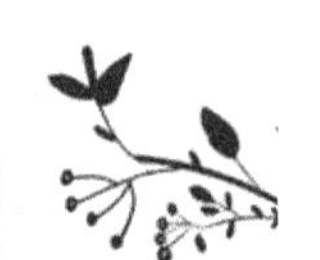

DAILY MEAL PLANNER

DATE: _______________________

M T W T F S S

BREAKFAST

GROCERY LIST

LUNCH

DINNER

NOTES

SNACKS

 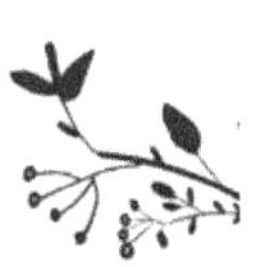

DAILY MEAL PLANNER

DATE _______________________________   M T W T F S S

BREAKFAST

GROCERY LIST

LUNCH

DINNER

NOTES

SNACKS

 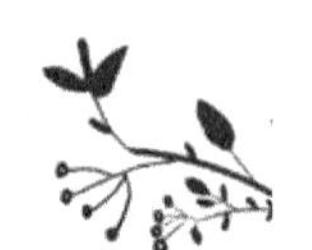

DAILY MEAL PLANNER

DATE: ___________________________   M T W T F S S

BREAKFAST

GROCERY LIST

LUNCH

DINNER

NOTES

SNACKS

DAILY MEAL PLANNER

DATE _______________   M T W T F S S

BREAKFAST	GROCERY LIST

BREAKFAST

LUNCH

DINNER

SNACKS

GROCERY LIST

NOTES

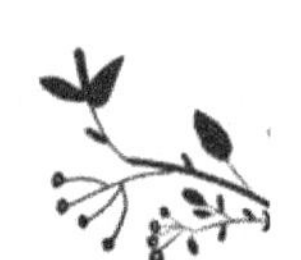

DAILY MEAL PLANNER

DATE: ___________________________   M T W T F S S

BREAKFAST

LUNCH

DINNER

SNACKS

GROCERY LIST

NOTES

DAILY MEAL PLANNER

DATE ___________________________   M T W T F S S

BREAKFAST

LUNCH

DINNER

SNACKS

GROCERY LIST

NOTES

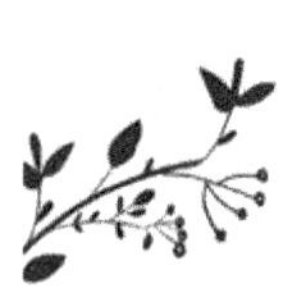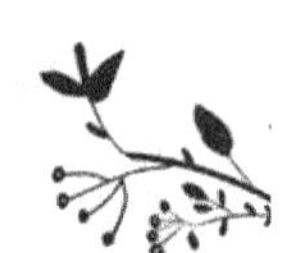

DAILY MEAL PLANNER

DATE: _______________________   M T W T F S S

BREAKFAST

GROCERY LIST

LUNCH

DINNER

NOTES

SNACKS

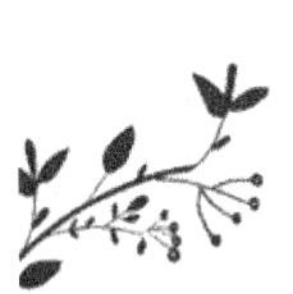

DAILY MEAL PLANNER

DATE _______________________   M T W T F S S

BREAKFAST

LUNCH

DINNER

SNACKS

GROCERY LIST

NOTES

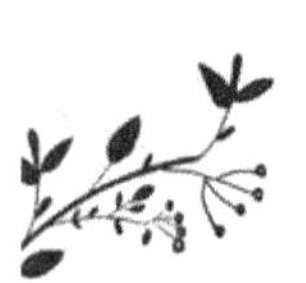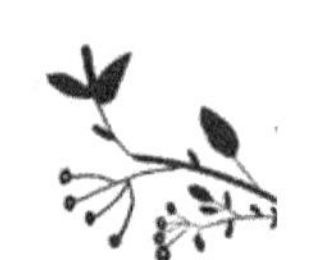

DAILY MEAL PLANNER

DATE: __________________________   M T W T F S S

BREAKFAST

GROCERY LIST

LUNCH

DINNER

NOTES

SNACKS

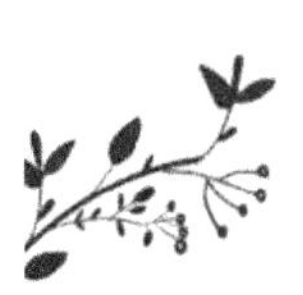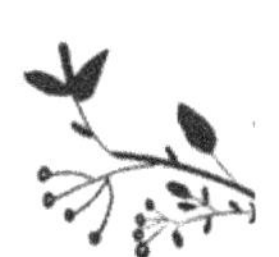

DAILY MEAL PLANNER

DATE ___________________________   M T W T F S S

BREAKFAST

LUNCH

DINNER

SNACKS

GROCERY LIST

NOTES

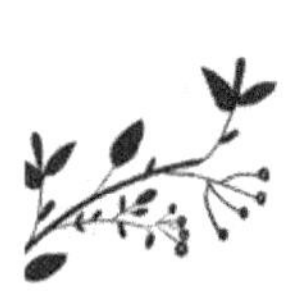 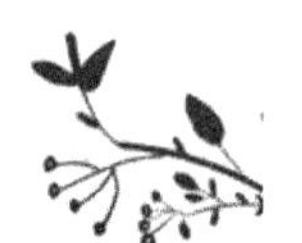

DAILY MEAL PLANNER

DATE: __________________________   M T W T F S S

BREAKFAST

LUNCH

DINNER

SNACKS

GROCERY LIST

NOTES

DAILY MEAL PLANNER

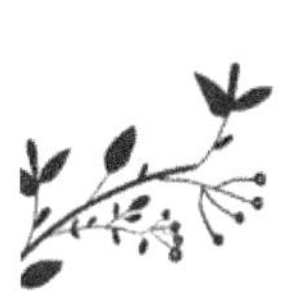

DATE ___________________________   M T W T F S S

BREAKFAST

GROCERY LIST

LUNCH

DINNER

NOTES

SNACKS

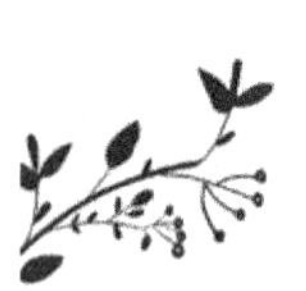 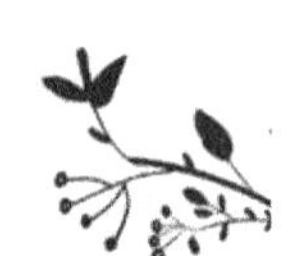

DAILY MEAL PLANNER

DATE: _______________________   M T W T F S S

BREAKFAST

LUNCH

DINNER

SNACKS

GROCERY LIST

NOTES

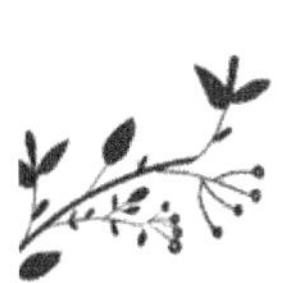

DAILY MEAL PLANNER

DATE ________________________   M T W T F S S

BREAKFAST

GROCERY LIST

LUNCH

DINNER

NOTES

SNACKS

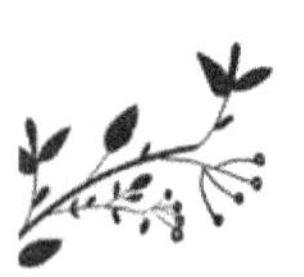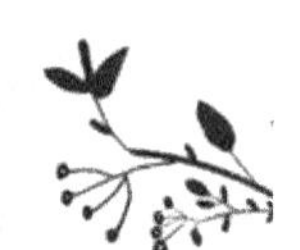

DAILY MEAL PLANNER

DATE: __________________________   M T W T F S S

BREAKFAST

GROCERY LIST

LUNCH

DINNER

NOTES

SNACKS

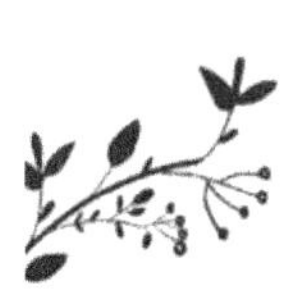

DAILY MEAL PLANNER

DATE _______________________   M T W T F S S

BREAKFAST

GROCERY LIST

LUNCH

DINNER

NOTES

SNACKS

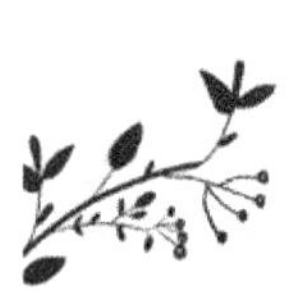 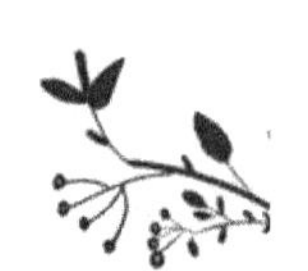

DAILY MEAL PLANNER

DATE ___________________________   M T W T F S S

BREAKFAST

LUNCH

DINNER

SNACKS

GROCERY LIST

NOTES

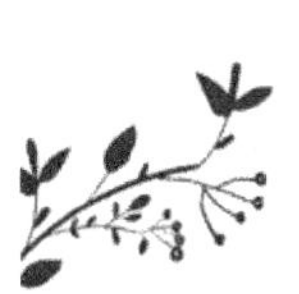

DAILY MEAL PLANNER

DATE: ___________________________   M T W T F S S

BREAKFAST

LUNCH

DINNER

SNACKS

GROCERY LIST

NOTES

 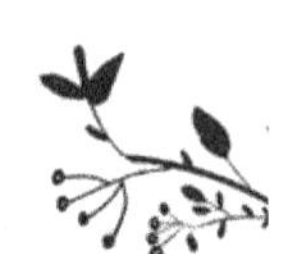

DAILY MEAL PLANNER

DATE: _______________________   M T W T F S S

BREAKFAST

GROCERY LIST

LUNCH

DINNER

NOTES

SNACKS

Acknowledgements

Thank you for taking the time to read this comprehensive guide to managing PCOS and Type 2 diabetes through diet, exercise, stress management, and more. We hope you found the information valuable and empowering as you embark on your journey towards a healthier, happier future.

This book would not have been possible without the invaluable contributions of our team of experts, who provided their expertise and insights to ensure the accuracy and relevance of the information presented. We are deeply grateful for their dedication to helping individuals manage these conditions effectively.

We also extend our sincerest gratitude to our readers, who we hope will find the information in this book helpful and motivating as they navigate the challenges of PCOS and Type 2 diabetes. Your willingness to learn and take control of your health is truly inspiring.

Thank you once again for reading!